EOSINOPHILIC
ESOPHAGITIS
COOKBOOK FOR KIDS

Deliciously Safe: Nourishing Recipes
Tailored for Kids with Eosinophilic
Esophagitis

Rhonda C. Anderson MS, RDN

Disclaimer

This cookbook's recipes and nutritional data are solely meant to be used for instructive and informative reasons. Despite our best efforts to assure accuracy, we advise you to speak with a certified healthcare provider or nutritionist before making any major dietary changes for your kid, particularly if they have special dietary needs, allergies, or other health issues.

This cookbook's writers and publishers disclaim all liability for any negative effects, harm, or losses brought on by using the recipes or information on this page.

When cooking meals for kids, parents and other caregivers are urged to use common sense and discretion while keeping in mind each child's unique dietary requirements and preferences. To further assure safety and prevent mishaps, adult supervision is recommended when youngsters are handling ingredients or cooking. These terms are acknowledged and accepted when you use this cookbook.

<u>Dedication</u>

This cookbook is dedicated with love to all the children who heroically fight eosinophilic esophagitis (EoE) around the world, as well as to their supporters. We are daily inspired by your bravery and tenacity, tough individuals overcoming the obstacles of the End of the Earth. Your resolute nature radiates, shedding light on the way for those facing comparable challenges.

You inspire us with your incredible fortitude and tenacity in the face of hardship, serving as a constant reminder of the strength of hope and endurance. This cookbook, which offers scrumptious and nourishing meals catered to your specific dietary requirements, should be a source of inspiration and solace. Recognize that you are not traveling alone on this road; instead, you are surrounded by kind people who want the best for you and your accomplishment. We stand with you together, unified in our determination to provide compassionate, empathetic, and loving support to one another.

Table of Contents

Introduction

Seven-year-old Mikel Kobbs battled a chronic immune system disease called Eosinophilic Esophagitis (EoE), which causes inflammation of the esophagus, for several months. Despite his young, Mikel had emotional and psychological side effects in addition to physical ones.

Since Mikel's grandma, with whom he resided, was unaware of it for an extended period of time, his health deteriorated. Mikel kept his severe chest pain and difficulty swallowing to himself until his parents paid him an unexpected visit.

Following a series of tests, the definitive diagnosis was eosinophilic esophagitis. When they heard of this, Mikel's parents were devastated since they were unsure of what lay ahead and worried for their son's safety.

When they sought counsel from a trustworthy family friend, she recommended seeking professional assistance. At that moment, I stepped in and provided them with a detailed plan that was tailored to Mikel's dietary needs utilizing the "Eosinophilic Esophagitis Cookbook for Kids."

Armed with healthful recipes and expert advice, Mikel's parents embarked on a mission to heal their child. With dedication and perseverance, they witnessed amazing progress as Mikel began to recover and gain energy.

Their heartfelt gratitude and stories of Mikel's speedy recuperation attest to the cookbook's effectiveness and the significance of a nutritious diet in avoiding EoE.

Finally, if you're a parent going through similar struggles, know that you're not alone. Investing in this invaluable resource is a crucial initial step in restoring your child's health and well-being.

I can assure you that if you implement the suggestions in this book, not only will your child grow, but you will also advocate for its use and help others who are in need.

This is the moment to set your child up for success in the future. Flip through the pages of the "Eosinophilic Esophagitis Cookbook for Kids" to unlock the key to healing and hope.

Chapter 1

Understanding Eosinophilic Esophagitis

What is Eosinophilic Esophagitis

Eosinophilic esophagitis is a long-term immune-system illness that occurs. This illness causes an accumulation of eosinophils, a type of white blood cell, in the tube lining the opening between your mouth and stomach. The esophagus is another name for this tube. This accumulation, which is brought on by certain foods, allergies, or acid reflux, can damage or inflame the tissue that lines the esophagus. Food may become caught in your throat or become difficult to swallow if you have damaged esophageal tissue.

Although it has only been recognized since the early 1990s, eosinophilic esophagitis is currently recognized as a significant contributor to digestive system disorders. Current research is expected to result in modifications to the diagnosis and management of eosinophilic esophagitis.

Diagnosis & Treatment

How Is Eosinophilic Esophagitis Diagnosed?

Currently, an upper endoscopy to check for esophageal inflammation is the only accurate method of diagnosing eosinophilic esophagitis. Your child's physician will take biopsies, or tiny samples of tissue, during the upper endoscopy to search for eosinophils, a particular kind of inflammatory cell. Eosinophilic esophagitis may be indicated if there are more than 15 eosinophils and other inflammatory causes, such as gastric reflux, have been ruled out.

How Is Eosinophilic Esophagitis Treated?

Physicians usually use medication, dietary modifications, or both to treat eosinophilic esophagitis.

Dietary modification

Even though eosinophilic esophagitis is a chronic ailment, most affected individuals can completely eradicate their symptoms by avoiding the foods that cause them. Dietary therapy can be approached in three primary ways: adhering to a rigorous elemental diet, eliminating foods as suggested by the allergy test, or avoiding the foods identified by the test.

avoiding the items that the allergy test recommended. Using this method, your child stays away from three to six foods for which their allergy test results were positive. About 50 to 75 percent of individuals have relief from eosinophilic esophagitis symptoms with this method, as allergy testing are not always reliable.

Empirical food elimination diet.

Your child follows this diet by avoiding foods including dairy, eggs, wheat, and soy that are known to be the most prevalent allergens.

Strict elemental diet.

Under this diet, your child's entire nutritional intake comes from a specially formulated combination of lipids, carbohydrates, amino acids, vitamins, and minerals. Usually, this diet starts with a complete food restriction, and then items are progressively added back in until medical professionals identify which foods are triggering your child's allergic responses.

<u>**This approach has a 95 percent success rate**</u>.

In order to provide optimal nutrition for children and adults following an elemental diet, we may utilize a special tube known as a "G-tube" to administer the formula straight into your child's stomach. It may be necessary to give nourishment straight into the bloodstream in really serious situations.

<u>Medication</u>

Using medicine is another strategy for managing eosinophilic esophagitis. Topical steroids, acid-blocking medications such proton pump inhibitors, or both are frequently used in this situation. Your child's doctor can assist you in weighing the benefits and drawbacks of using drugs to treat the illness vs following a restricted diet.

Causes & Triggers

Different cells assemble during an allergic reaction to produce symptoms like redness, swelling, and itching. One kind of white blood cell responsible for an allergic reaction is the eosinophil.

Eosinophils are a vital component of the immune system that are constantly present in trace amounts in the blood and intestine, where they combat parasites and carry out other tasks. But when eosinophils proliferate in organs other than the intestine and blood, they become problematic.

Eosinophils are found in your nose if you have seasonal allergies, in your lungs if you have asthma, and in your esophagus if you have EoE.

Children with eosinophilic esophagitis can be found across all ethnic groups and financial brackets. Children with eoe frequently suffer from eczema, seasonal allergies, or asthma in addition to other allergic illnesses.

Three decades prior, EoE was unheard of. Over the last five years, there has been a sharp increase in diagnoses. We are unsure if this is because more people are actually recognizing the sickness, or if it is indeed getting more common. Most likely, a combination of the two variables is to blame for the increasing number of cases. With an estimated occurrence rate of 1 in 1,500 children, EoE remains an uncommon illness.

What Causes Eosinophilic Esophagitis In Children?

eosinophilic Food allergies are the most common cause of esophagitis, an allergic condition.

The most frequently mentioned foods in relation to eosinophilic esophagitis are dairy products and milk, wheat, eggs, soy, peanuts, tree nuts, fish, and shellfish.

Symptoms In Children

Children who have eosinophilic esophagitis experience esophageal swelling and inflammation. Symptoms of the inflammation can include food impaction, vomiting, and pain during feedings.

While every child's symptoms may vary, the following are typical indications of eosinophilic esophagitis:

1.Difficulty feeding, in infants

2.Difficulty eating, in children

3.Vomiting

4.Abdominal pain

5.Difficulty swallowing, also called dysphagia

6.Food getting stuck in the esophagus after swallowing, also known as impaction

7.No response to GERD medication

8.Failure to thrive, including poor growth, malnutrition and weight loss

It's crucial to keep in mind that several of these symptoms might coexist with other illnesses, such as gastroesophageal reflux disease, and that none of them clearly indicate eosinophilic esophagitis. Eosinophilic esophagitis can affect healthy children and adults, but it is more common in children with other allergy diseases (including asthma, eczema, and traditional food allergies). For this reason, it's critical that your child receives a diagnosis from experts who have extensive knowledge of pediatric eosinophilic esophagitis.

Chapter 2

The Role of Diet in Managing Eosinophilic Esophagitis

How Diet Affects Eosinophilic Esophagitis

When it comes to treating children's Eosinophilic Esophagitis (EoE), diet is vital. Some foods may assist treat EoE symptoms, while others may exacerbate the illness by causing inflammation in the esophagus. Parents and other caregivers can make wise decisions for their children's health if they are aware of how diet influences early onset of epilepsy (EoE).

1.Determining Trigger meals: Determining trigger meals that exacerbate symptoms is one of the first steps in managing eating disorders. Dairy, wheat, soy, eggs, nuts, and seafood are common triggers. Maintaining a food diary facilitates the identification of potential trigger foods, enabling efficient elimination.

2. Elemental Diet: If a kid's allergies are severe, an elemental diet may be advised, in which case the youngster only drinks formula based on amino acids and all probable allergens are eliminated. This method can be quite successful in relieving the discomfort and promoting esophageal healing.

3. Elimination Diets: In order to identify which food groups or allergens are causing inflammation, elimination diets include eliminating them from the diet. It is essential to collaborate with a dietician or healthcare professional to make sure the youngster is getting enough nutrients and stays away from trigger foods.

4. Allergy Testing: Specific food allergies that may be causing EoE can be found using allergy testing methods like skin prick or blood tests. A child's individualized food plan can be developed with their sensitivities in mind.

5. Texture Modifications: Food texture can be changed to help children with EoE swallow food more easily and have less esophageal irritation. This may entail choosing softer, smoother foods over ones with scratchy or coarse textures.

6. Slow Food Introduction: Once trigger foods have been identified, reintroducing them one at a time in little amounts might assist ascertain whether they still elicit symptoms. This incremental strategy can identify particular triggers and direct long-term dietary management.

7.Nutritional Support: It's critical to make sure the child has enough nourishment even on a restricted diet. Creating meal plans with the assistance of a dietitian can help ensure that the child's nutritional needs are met and that their growth and development are supported.

8.Family Support and Education: It can be difficult for families to manage eating disorders through nutrition. Making the process easier and less stressful for caregivers can be achieved by educating and supporting them on how to manage dietary restrictions, label reading, and meal preparation.

9. Monitoring and Modifying: It's essential to schedule routine check-ins with medical professionals in order to keep an eye on the child's development and alter the diet plan as needed. This continuous assistance can improve EoE management tactics.

Creating a Safe Food Environment for Kids

Dear Parents,

Establishing a safe eating environment becomes critical if your child is diagnosed with eosinophilic esophagitis. This disease involves esophageal inflammation, and some foods may have negative side effects. Here are some useful advice to make sure your child is safe:

1. Recognizing Food Triggers: Be mindful of the foods that can set off symptoms. To track responses, maintain a food journal. Collaborate with your child's medical team to determine possible triggers.

2. Reading Labels: Pay close attention to food labels when you go grocery shopping to steer clear of allergies or substances that could aggravate eosinophilic esophagitis. Select foods with ingredient lists that are easy to read and understand.

3.Cooking from Scratch: If you want more control over the ingredients, think about preparing meals yourself. By doing this, you can stay away from preservatives and substances that might have negative effects.

4.Educating Family Members: Make sure your child's food limitations and condition are known to your family members. A clear line of communication can help avoid unintentional exposure to trigger foods.

5.Establishing a Secure Area: Assign particular sections of the kitchen and pantry to the secure keeping of food suitable for individuals with allergies. This will lessen the possibility of cross-contamination.

6. Meal Planning: Arrange your meals in advance to guarantee a balanced and allergy-free diet for your youngster. To make meals fun and nourishing, get creative with your recipe writing.

7. Including Your Child: Let your kids help with meal preparation and planning. They learn about their nutritional requirements from this, and it also gives them the confidence to choose foods wisely.

8.Seek Assistance: Establish contact with internet forums or support organizations for parents of kids suffering from eosinophilic esophagitis. Navigating this condition can be made much easier by exchanging experiences and advice.

9. Working with Medical Professionals: Make sure your child is receiving the right care and that their condition is being monitored for any changes by scheduling regular consultations with allergists and nutritionists, among other medical professionals.

10. Highlighting Little Wins: Keep in mind to acknowledge and cherish the minor triumphs your child has experienced while coping with eosinophilic esophagitis. Any successful meal that doesn't cause any negative reactions is a positive step.

You may provide a secure and encouraging eating environment for your child who has eosinophilic esophagitis by implementing these methods. Recall that you can support your child's success despite the difficulties this condition presents if you have the necessary patience, persistence, and resources.

Questions and Answers

Question 1
What Age Does Eosinophilic Esophagitis Occur?

Answer

While young people in their third or fourth decade of life, as well as school-age children (6–12), are usually affected by eosinophilic esophagitis. 16 It may also exist in infants under the age of one year.

Question 2

What is the First line Treatment For Eosinophilic Esophagitis?

Answer

It's crucial to remember that the US Food and Drug Administration has not yet approved any medical treatments for EoE. Using corticosteroids topically Once an Eoe diagnosis is confirmed, topical corticosteroids are often utilized as first line medicines and are the cornerstone of treatment for the condition.

Question 3.

How common is eosinophilic esophagitis (EoE)?

Answer

In the US, the estimated number of patients with EoE is 55 per 100,000 individuals. Depending on the area, this could change.

Question 4.

Was my child born with EoE?

Answer

It is unlikely that children are born with EoE; instead, it develops over time. It's possible that they are predisposed to the illness from birth.

Question 5.

Is it harmful if someone only has a few eosinophils in their esophagus?

Answer

It is possible that there is esophageal inflammation based on the presence of eosinophils. It's important to address inflammation whenever it occurs and not to neglect it. It is yet unknown, though, how many eosinophils are "too many" and how long is "too long."

Question 6
What are the symptoms of EoE in infants?

Answer
The symptoms of reflux that infants with EoE typically experience include spitting up, irritability, vomiting, and unwillingness to eat. Some kids could also struggle with their growth.

Question 7
What are the symptoms of EoE in toddlers?

Answer
Toddlers with EoE may also experience difficulty transitioning to solid foods or complain of abdominal

pain, while their symptoms are similar to those of newborns.

Question 8

What are the symptoms of EoE in school-aged children?

Answer

Children at school may experience symptoms similar to reflux and occasionally throw up. They might have trouble swallowing, but they might find it difficult to articulate this.

Question 9

What are symptoms of EoE in older children and teens?

Answer

In addition to the symptoms seen in the other age groups, older children and teens may additionally complain of trouble swallowing or food being lodged in their esophagus.

Question 10
Who should be tested for EoE?

Answer
Patients who do not react to medical treatment and have symptoms indicated at the top of this page may be tested for EoE. This is particularly true for people who have severe trouble swallowing solid food.

Question 11.
Is EoE hereditary?

Answer
EoE might run in families more frequently. If a family member exhibits symptoms, testing should be done.

Question 12.

Do children outgrow EoE?

Answer

Data about the long-term effects of EoE are scarce.

Question 13.

Can inflammation of the esophagus be cancerous?

Answer

Although there is insufficient data to make a firm conclusion, inflammation may not cause cancer, according to limited adult research. Any inflammatory process that continues into adulthood from childhood needs to be taken seriously.

Question 14.

What happens if someone with an eosinophilic disorder is exposed to an "unsafe" food?

Answer

EoE responses might not occur right away. Generally speaking, a child's symptoms may worsen in a matter of days if they are exposed to a "unsafe" food.

Question 15.

Is it true that some children with EoE cannot eat food?

Answer

While most kids with EoE can consume some food, each patient is a little bit different. For their nourishment, certain patients are compelled to use specially formulated formulations. We refer to these diet plans as elemental diets. Find out more about the various diets that are used to get rid of EoE symptoms.

Chapter 3

Essential Kitchen Tools and Ingredients

Must-Have Kitchen Tools for EOE-Friendly Cooking

1. Food Scale: Helpful for accurately measuring ingredients in EOE-friendly recipes.

2. Blender: Great for blending foods safe for the environment to make sauces, soups, and smoothies.

3. Food processor: excellent for combining, pureeing, and cutting items that are acceptable for EOE.

4. Steamer: Useful for maintaining the nutrients in meats and veggies while they cook.

5. Rice Cooker: Ideal for cooking grains that are frequently EOE-friendly, such quinoa and rice.

6. Immersion Blender: Useful for mixing little amounts of sauces and soups right in pots.

7. Silicone Baking Mats: You may bake EOE-safe sweets without greasiness in your pans by using these non-stick mats.

8. Stainless Steel Cookware: For cooking that is EOE-friendly, cookware that is sturdy and non-reactive is a must.

9. Airtight Food Storage Containers: Avoid cross-contamination and maintain the freshness of EOE-safe foods.

10. Cutting boards: To prevent allergy contamination, keep separate ones for foods that are OK for EOE.

11.The vegetable spiralizer is a helpful tool for making gluten-free vegetable noodles.

12. Citrus Juicer: Use the fresh juice of citrus fruits to flavor foods that are safe for the environment.

13. Oven Thermometer: Make sure you bake EOE-friendly meals at the right temperature.

14. Measuring Cups and Spoons: These are necessary to measure ingredients precisely while cooking in an EOE-safe manner.

15. Instant-Read Thermometer: Verify that meats are cooked safely by taking their internal temperature.

16. Mandoline Slicer: Use this culinary equipment to rapidly and evenly slice fruits and vegetables.

17. Nut Milk Bag: For EOE-safe drinks, strain homemade nut milks or juices.

18. Herb Keeper: To improve the flavors of meals that are EOE-friendly, keep herbs fresh for longer.

19. Microplane Zester: Finely grate materials for flavor enhancement after extracting zest from citrus fruits.

20. Salad Spinner: Completely dry fresh produce for salads and other foods that are good for the environment.

Key Ingredients for Delicious and Nutritious Meals

Making tasty and nourishing meals for children with eosinophilic esophagitis requires careful consideration of which important ingredients are healthy and flavorful, as well as meeting their unique dietary requirements.

Caregivers may easily make pleasant meals that not only accommodate the dietary limitations connected with the condition but also encourage general well-being by incorporating a variety of healthful and allergen-friendly items. Let's examine some essential components that can be used to make tasty and healthful meals for kids suffering from eosinophilic esophagitis.

1. Lean Proteins: Adding lean proteins to meals is key for supplying vital nutrients and promoting children's healthy growth and development. Choose protein-rich, easier-to-digest foods like skinless chicken, fish, tofu, and lentils if you have eosinophilic esophagitis.

2. Whole Grains: Rich in fiber, vitamins, and minerals, whole grains are a great source of nutrition. Select foods like millet, quinoa, brown rice, and gluten-free oats to provide meals some texture and variation while still giving the kids a healthy amount of energy.

3. Fruits and Vegetables: Adding a rainbow of colors to foods not only makes them seem better, but it also gives them vital vitamins, minerals, and antioxidants. To reduce the risk of irritating the esophagus, use softer types such as mashed sweet potatoes, boiled carrots, bananas, and applesauce.

4. Healthy Fats: To promote brain function and general health, include sources of healthy fats such avocados, olive oil, nuts, and seeds. These fats aid in the body's reduction of inflammation and aid in the absorption of fat-soluble vitamins.

5. Dairy Substitutes: When preparing dishes that call for conventional dairy products, parents of children with eosinophilic esophagitis who are sensitive to dairy products can think about substituting dairy with almond, coconut, or oat milk. These substitutes may be less uncomfortable while still providing vital minerals like calcium and vitamin D.

6. Herbs and Spices: Instead of utilizing components that can cause symptoms, enhance the flavor profile of meals with herbs and spices. In addition to giving food depth, fresh herbs like basil, parsley, and chives and spices like turmeric, ginger, and cinnamon have anti-inflammatory qualities.

7. Allergen-Free Ingredients: When cooking, keep in mind common allergens including wheat, eggs, peanuts, tree nuts, and soy. Make sure the ingredients are safe for kids with eosinophilic esophagitis by carefully reading food labels or choosing allergen-free options.

8. Hydration: Throughout the day, provide water and herbal teas to promote proper hydration. Maintaining enough hydration levels helps support healthy digestion and esophageal function.

Thoughtfully and creatively combining these essential ingredients allows caregivers to provide a range of delicious and nourishing meals that meet the specific nutritional needs of kids suffering with eosinophilic esophagitis.

A well-rounded and pleasurable dining experience can be provided while promoting the general wellbeing of these young people by experimenting with various recipes and including a varied selection of foods.

Always remember to speak with a medical professional or a qualified dietitian for individualized nutritional advice and recommendations catered to your child's unique requirements.

Chapter 4

Safe Breakfast Recipes

Morning Meals for Happy Tummies

1.Berry oatmeal Muffins.

Berries that are in season are highlighted in these moist muffins. Try blackberries and raspberries as well, or a combo of both.

Prep Time: 15mins

Cook Time: 20 mins
Servings: 12

Ingredients

- ¾ cup quick cooking oats
- ¼ cup wheat germ
- 1 ½ cups all-purpose flour
- ½ cup sugar
- ½ cup chopped walnuts
- ½ teaspoon salt
- 1 tablespoon baking powder
- ¾ cup milk
- ½ cup vegetable oil
- 1 egg
- 1 cup blueberries
- ⅓ cup quick cooking oats
- ¼ cup brown sugar
- 1 teaspoon ground cinnamon

Directions

1. Set oven temperature to 400 F, or 200 C. Grease 12 muffin tins very lightly.

2. Combine the flour, sugar, walnuts, baking powder, wheat germ, and 3/4 cup of oats in a big basin. Just until the dry ingredients are evenly moistened, stir in the egg, oil, and milk. Add the blueberries and fold. Pour batter into muffin tins that have been prepped.

3. In a separate bowl, combine 1/3 cup oats, cinnamon, and brown sugar; sprinkle over batter.

4. Place the muffins in the preheated oven and bake for 20 minutes, or until a knife inserted into the center of the muffin comes out clean.

Nutritional Fact

277 calories, 14g Fat, 35g carbs, 5g protein.

2.Peanut Butter Banana Smoothie

This smoothie with peanut butter and banana is delicious and refreshing.

Prep Time: 5 mins
Servings:4

Ingredients

- 2 bananas, broken into chunks
- 2 cups milk
- ½ cup peanut butter
- 2 tablespoons honey, or to taste
- 2 cups ice cubes

Directions

1. Compile the ingredients.
2. In a blender, combine the bananas, milk, peanut butter, honey, and ice cubes.
3. Blend for about 30 seconds, or until smooth.
4. Present and savor.

3.Blueberry Lemon Breakfast Quinoa

In this oatmeal substitute, sharp lemon and sweet blueberries work well together. Quinoa, which is high in fiber and protein, makes a fantastic breakfast. One morning, my adorable kid Ferdinand was hungry quinoa and wanted something different from what he usually had, so I made this up. To thin, pour additional milk over top. Good with a dash of nutmeg or cinnamon as well.

Prep Time:5 mins
Cook Time:25 mins
Servings: 2

Ingredients
- 1 cup quinoa
- 2 cups nonfat milk
- 1 pinch salt
- 3 tablespoons maple syrup
- ½ lemon, zested
- 1 cup blueberries
- 2 teaspoons flax seed

Directions

1. To get rid of the bitterness, rinse the quinoa in a fine strainer with cold water until the water flows clear and isn't foamy.

2. In a saucepan over medium heat, warm the milk for two to three minutes. After adding the quinoa and salt to the milk, simmer it over medium-low heat for about 20 minutes, or until most of the liquid has been absorbed. Take the pot off of the burner. Incorporate the lemon zest and maple syrup into the quinoa mixture. Fold blueberries into mixture gently.

3. Spoon quinoa mixture into each of two dishes; garnish with 1 tsp flax seed to serve.

4.Chia Seed Pudding

A tasty and nutritious way for your child to begin the day or end it.

Prep Time:15 mins
Servings:4
Additional Time:8 hrs 30 mins.

Ingredients

- 1 cup unsweetened vanilla-flavored almond milk
- 1 cup vanilla fat-free yogurt
- 2 tablespoons pure maple syrup
- 1 teaspoon pure vanilla extract
- ⅛ teaspoon salt
- ¼ cup chia seeds
- 1 pint strawberries, hulled and chopped
- 4 teaspoons pure maple syrup
- ¼ cup toasted almonds

Directions

1. In a dish, whisk together almond milk, yogurt, two tablespoons maple syrup, vanilla, and salt until just combined. Add the chia seeds, whisk to mix them in, and let them soak for half an hour.
2. To disperse the seeds that have collected throughout the mixture, stir the chia seed mixture. Place plastic wrap over the bowl and chill for eight hours or overnight.

3. Place 4 teaspoons of maple syrup in a bowl with the strawberries and toss to coat. Stir the strawberries with the almonds.

4. Divide the chia seed mixture into four bowls and place some of the strawberry mixture on top of each.

5.Rice Cake

These rice cakes are usually served for breakfast, but sometimes I have them for dinner when my husband is away and I want to make something simple and quick for the kids. Every time we had leftover rice in the refrigerator when I was a child, I remember my dad cooking them for me. Topped with salsa, they taste amazing! This is a wonderful starting recipe that can be easily customized to suit the needs of any child with eosinophilic esophagitis.

Prep Time:5 mins
Cook Time: 5 mins
Servings: 1

Ingredients

- ½ cup cooked white rice
- 1 egg
- 1 tablespoon chopped fresh basil (Optional)
- 1 teaspoon milk
- salt and ground black pepper to taste
- 1 ½ teaspoons butter

Directions

1. In a bowl, combine rice, egg, basil, milk, salt, and pepper.
2. In a skillet over medium heat, melt butter. Transfer half of the rice mixture into each of the two skillets. Cook for about 3 minutes, or until the bottom is browned. After flipping, heat for a further two minutes, or until the second side is browned.

6.Quinoa Porridge

Prep Time:5 mins
Cook Time: 30 mins
Servings: 3

Ingredients

- ½ cup quinoa
- ¼ teaspoon ground cinnamon
- 1 ½ cups almond milk
- ½ cup water
- 2 tablespoons brown sugar
- 1 teaspoon vanilla extract (Optional)
- 1 pinch salt

Directions

1. Add the quinoa to a pot that has been heated to medium heat. Add cinnamon for seasoning and cook, stirring often, until toasted, about 3 minutes. After adding the water, vanilla, and almond milk,

whisk in the salt and brown sugar. After bringing to a boil, reduce the heat and simmer for about 25 minutes, or until the porridge is thick and the grains are soft. If the liquid has dried up before the food is done cooking, add more water as needed. Stir from time to time, especially toward the end, to avoid scorching.

7. Vegetables Birdseed Pilaf

a tasty millet and vegetable pilaf spiced with wine and rosemary for vegetarians. I gave it the goofy title since my daughter thought it was so cute that it was constructed with "birdseed." Add more freshly grated Parmesan cheese to the dish.

Prep Time: 10 mins
Cook Time: 40 mins
Servings: 6

Ingredients

- 1 ¼ cups millet, rinsed and drained

- 2 ½ cups vegetable broth
- 1 tablespoon olive oil
- 1 onion, chopped
- 6 cloves garlic, minced
- 1 (10 ounce) package frozen chopped spinach
- 1 cup frozen peas
- ¾ cup white wine
- 1 teaspoon minced fresh rosemary
- 4 plum tomatoes, chopped
- salt and ground black pepper to taste
- ½ cup grated Parmesan cheese

Directions

1. In a large saucepan over medium heat, cook and stir the millet for 5 to 8 minutes, or until aromatic and toasted.

2. In a big saucepan, bring the vegetable broth to a boil. Then, add the millet and bring it back to a boil. Once the liquid has been absorbed, reduce heat to medium-low, cover the saucepan, and simmer for 18 to 22 minutes.

3. In a skillet over medium heat, heat the olive oil. Cook and stir the onion and garlic for 5 to 10 minutes, or until the onion is transparent.

4. Add wine and rosemary to the millet and whisk in the onion combination, spinach, and peas. Turn the heat up to medium, cover the pan, and cook for seven to ten minutes, stirring now and then. Add the tomatoes, salt, and pepper; cover again and cook for 2 to 3 minutes, or until the tomatoes are tender. After taking the pot off the stove, mix the millet mixture with Parmesan cheese.

Tips

Add more wine at the end of cooking if the millet mixture is too dry.

8.Polenta with Tomato sauce

This quick and simple dish for polenta with tomato sauce is a hit with my kids. The next day and the day after that too are excellent for eating leftovers! If desired, sprinkle more Parmesan cheese over top.

Prep Time: 10 mins

Cook Time: 20 mins

Servings: 6

Ingredients

- 2 cups milk
- 2 cups chicken stock
- 1 cup yellow cornmeal
- 1 cup Parmesan cheese
- 2 cups spaghetti sauce

Directions

1. Set the oven's temperature to 350°F, or 175°C. Coat a 9-inch baking dish with grease.

2. Fill a big saucepan with milk and chicken stock and heat it to a rolling boil over medium-high heat. Stir in cornmeal gradually, being careful not to create lumps. Simmer until thick, stirring regularly, for around five minutes, after reducing the heat to low. Take off the heat and add the Parmesan cheese.

3. Spoon spaghetti sauce over the polenta that has been prepared in the baking dish.

4. Bake for 10 minutes or until the sauce is bubbling in the preheated oven.

<u>Tips</u>
Make use of your preferred spaghetti sauce.

9.Savory Sweet Potato Hash

Prep Time: 10 mins.
Cook Time: 15 mins.
Servings: 2.

Ingredients
- 1 large sweet potato, diced
- 1 tablespoon water, or as needed
- salt to taste
- 1 tablespoon olive oil
- 1 small white onion, diced
- 1 cup diced ham steak
- ¼ teaspoon ground cinnamon
- ¼ teaspoon cayenne pepper

- 1 teaspoon brown sugar, or to taste

Directions

1. Add water and salt to a microwave-safe bowl with the sweet potato. After two to three minutes in the microwave, somewhat soften; drain.

2. In a skillet over medium heat, heat the olive oil; sauté and toss the onion for 3 to 4 minutes, or until it softens slightly. Add sweet potato, ham, cinnamon, cayenne, and salt to onion; place a lid on the skillet. Add the brown sugar and heat, stirring periodically, until the sweet potatoes are cooked through, about 10 minutes. For one to two more minutes, cook and stir until the brown sugar is dissolved.

10.Perfect Summer Fruit Salad

Prep Time: 25 mins
Cook Time: 5 mins

Additional Time: 3 hrs 30 minutes
Servings: 10

Ingredients

Sauce
- ⅔ cup fresh orange juice
- ⅓ cup fresh lemon juice
- ⅓ cup packed brown sugar
- ½ teaspoon grated orange zest
- ½ teaspoon grated lemon zest
- 1 teaspoon vanilla extract

Salad
- 2 cups cubed fresh pineapple
- 2 cups strawberries, hulled and sliced
- 3 kiwi fruit, peeled and sliced
- 3 bananas, sliced
- 2 oranges, peeled and sectioned
- 1 cup seedless grapes
- 2 cups blueberries

Directions

To make the sauce, place a pot over medium-high heat and add the orange juice, lemon juice, brown sugar, orange zest, and lemon zest. Bring to a boil. Remove from heat and mix in vanilla essence. Reduce heat to medium-low and simmer until slightly thickened, about 5 minutes. Put aside to cool.

2. To make the salad, arrange the following fruits in a big, transparent glass bowl: bananas, oranges, grapes, pineapple, strawberries, and blueberries. Cover and chill the fruit for three to four hours before serving it with the chilled sauce on top.

11.Tofu Breakfast Burrito Bowls

Prep Time: 15 mins
Cook Time: 30 mins
Total Time: 45 mins
Servings: 3

Ingredients
- 3 tablespoons olive oil, divided

- 1 (14 ounce) package extra-firm tofu, drained
- ½ teaspoon salt
- black pepper to taste
- 1 ½ teaspoons onion powder
- 1 ½ teaspoons garlic powder
- ½ teaspoon ground turmeric
- 1 tablespoon fresh lemon juice
- 1 tablespoon olive oil
- 1 cup finely diced red onion
- 2 jalapeno peppers, seeded and chopped
- ½ teaspoon salt
- 3 cloves garlic, minced
- 2 cups chopped tomatoes
- 1 ½ teaspoons cumin
- ¼ cup chopped fresh cilantro
- 1 tablespoon fresh lemon juice
- 1 (15.5 ounce) can no-salt-added black beans, drained and rinsed
- 1 ½ cups cooked hash brown potatoes
- 1 avocado - peeled, pitted and sliced
- 1 teaspoon fresh lemon juice
- ¼ cup chopped fresh cilantro
- 1 teaspoon hot sauce, or to taste

Directions

1. Turn the heat to medium-high and preheat a large, heavy skillet. Put in two tablespoons of oil. Slice the tofu into bite-sized pieces over the skillet, season with salt and pepper, and heat, tossing constantly with a thin metal spatula, until the liquid evaporates and the tofu turns brown—about ten minutes. (If you see liquid accumulating in the pan, turn up the heat to help the water evaporate.) When stirring, be sure to get under the tofu to scrape up the crispy bits from the bottom of the pan and prevent them from sticking.

2. Add the juice, turmeric, onion and garlic powders, and the last tablespoon of oil, tossing to coat. Cook for an additional five minutes.

3. Turn up the heat to medium-high in a saucepan with a heavy bottom. Pour in some oil. Saute the onion and jalapeños for around five minutes, while stirring and adding a pinch of salt. Add the garlic

and stir-fry for about 30 seconds, or until fragrant. Stir in tomatoes, cumin, and remaining salt. Cook, stirring, for about 5 minutes, or until tomatoes are saucy. Add the lemon juice and cilantro. Allow cilantro to soften. Add the beans and cook for about two minutes, stirring now and again. Taste for seasoning and salt.

4. Transfer a small amount of hash browns, beans, and scramble into each bowl. Add avocado, cilantro, and a squeeze of fresh lemon juice on top. Accompany with spicy sauce.

12.Summer Berry Parfait With Yoghurt and Granola

This recipe makes a flexible parfait that can be enjoyed by children who have eosinophilic esophagitis. When cut in half, it makes a filling snack or a healthy breakfast. Although frozen blueberries work well, fresh strawberries are recommended.

Prep Time: 10 mins
Total Time: 10 mins
Servings: 1

Ingredients

- ¾ cup sliced strawberries
- ¾ cup blueberries
- 1 (6 ounce) container vanilla yogurt
- 1 tablespoon wheat germ
- ½ banana, sliced
- ⅓ cup granola

Directions

In a big bowl, arrange 1/4 cup blueberries, 1/4 cup strawberries, 1/3 container yogurt, 1/3 tablespoon wheat germ, 1/3 of the sliced banana, and around 2 tablespoons of granola. Once every ingredient has been utilized, keep layering the parfait and building it up.

13.Banana Pancakes

Easy and delicious homemade banana pancakes provide kids with eosinophilic esophagitis with a playful twist. They're a tasty treat that's simple to prepare from home and can be enjoyed in minutes.

Prep Time: 5 mins
Cook Time: 10 mins
Total Time: 15 mins
Servings: 6

Ingredients

- 1 cup all-purpose flour
- 1 tablespoon white sugar
- 2 teaspoons baking powder
- ¼ teaspoon salt
- 1 egg, beaten
- 1 cup milk
- 2 tablespoons vegetable oil
- 2 ripe bananas, mashed

Directions

1. Compile the ingredients.

2. In a bowl, mix flour, baking powder, white sugar, and salt. In a separate bowl, combine the egg, milk, vegetable oil, and bananas.

3. Stir the flour mixture into the banana mixture; a slightly lumpy batter will result.

4. Turn up the heat to medium-high and gently oil a frying pan or griddle. Using about 1/4 cup of batter for each pancake, pour or spoon the mixture onto the griddle.

5. Cook for 3 to 5 minutes on each side, or until pancakes are golden brown. Warm up the food.

6. Present warm and savor!

Chapter 5

Kid-Approved Lunch Ideas

1.Grilled Chicken Salad With Seasonal Fruit

Make a tasty and aesthetically pleasing grilled chicken salad with seasonal fruits, such as orange segments in winter and fresh berries in summer, for children with eosinophilic esophagitis.

Prep Time: 15 mins
Cook Time: 20 mins
Total Time: 35 mins
Servings: 6

Ingredients

- 1 pound skinless, boneless chicken breast halves
- ½ cup pecans
- ⅓ cup red wine vinegar
- ½ cup white sugar
- 1 cup vegetable oil
- ½ onion, minced
- 1 teaspoon ground mustard
- 1 teaspoon salt
- ¼ teaspoon ground white pepper
- 2 heads Bibb lettuce - rinsed, dried and torn
- 1 cup sliced fresh strawberries

Directions

1. Set the grill's temperature to high. Give the grill grate a little oil.
2. Grill chicken for about 8 minutes on each side, or until juices run clear. Take off the heat, let it cool, then cut. Put aside.

3. In the interim, toast pecans over medium-high heat in a dry skillet. Cook for about 8 minutes, stirring regularly, until pecans become aromatic. Take off the heat and place aside.

4. To prepare the dressing: In blender, combine red wine vinegar, sugar, vegetable oil, mustard, onion, salt, and pepper. Process till everything is smooth.

5. Place lettuce on platters for serving. Add pecans, strawberries, and slices of cooked chicken on top. To serve, drizzle with dressing.

2.South Western Quinoa Salad

Prep Time: 30 mins
Cook Time: 15 mins
Total Time: 45 mins
Servings: 8

Ingredients
- 1 cup quinoa
- 1 tablespoon butter
- 2 cups chicken broth
- ½ cup diced green bell pepper

- ½ cup diced red onion
- 1 cup corn
- 1 (15 ounce) can black beans, drained
- ¼ cup chopped cilantro
- 1 large tomato, diced
- ½ cup fresh lime juice, or to taste
- 2 tablespoons red wine vinegar
- 2 tablespoons olive oil
- 1 tablespoon adobo seasoning
- ½ cup feta cheese
- salt and black pepper to taste

Directions

1. Give the quinoa a good rinse in cold water and then drain.

2. In a big saucepan over medium heat, melt butter. Cook for about 3 minutes, stirring occasionally, or until water is gone and quinoa is lightly browned. Add the chicken broth and heat until it boils. After quinoa has absorbed stock, reduce heat to low and simmer for 10 minutes or so. Quinoa should be chilled for at least ten minutes in the fridge.

3. In a large salad bowl, combine green bell pepper, red onion, corn, black beans, cilantro, tomato, lime juice, red wine vinegar, olive oil, feta cheese, and adobo seasoning.

4. Gently mix in the quinoa and adjust the seasoning with extra lime juice, salt, and pepper to taste. Before serving, let salad cool for at least half an hour; serve cold.

3.Turkey Lettuce Wraps with Shiitake Mushrooms

Prep Time: 40 mins
Cook Time: 20 mins
Total Time: 60 mins
Servings: 4

Ingredients

- 2 cups water
- 2 ounces mai fun (angel hair) rice noodles

- 1 teaspoon vegetable oil
- 4 shiitake mushrooms, sliced
- 2 teaspoons vegetable oil
- 1 (16 ounce) package ground turkey
- 6 green onions, chopped
- ¼ cup chopped water chestnuts
- 4 teaspoons finely minced fresh ginger root
- 2 teaspoons minced garlic
- 3 tablespoons soy sauce
- 2 tablespoons brown sugar
- 1 tablespoon rice vinegar
- 1 teaspoon sesame oil
- 1 teaspoon finely grated orange zest
- 12 leaves green leaf lettuce

Toppings

- ½ cup bean sprouts
- 1 carrot, grated
- ½ cup salted peanuts
- ½ cup chopped fresh cilantro
- ½ cup sweet chili sauce

Directions

1.Place two cups of water in a small pot and bring to a boil. Once the heat is off, mix in the rice noodles. For five to seven minutes, cover and let the noodles soak until tender. Use cold water to rinse. Make sure to drain well.

2. In a large skillet over medium-high heat, heat 1 teaspoon of oil. For about two minutes, or until they are browned and tender, cook the mushrooms in the heated oil. Take the mushrooms out of the skillet. Hold back.

3. Warm up the pan's remaining two teaspoons of oil. For five to seven minutes, or until the turkey is no longer pink, cook and toss it in the oil. Add the garlic, ginger, water chestnuts, and green onions and sauté for an additional minute. Stir in brown sugar, soy sauce, and the saved mushrooms. For a short while, simmer to blend the flavors. Remove the pan from the heat and mix in the orange zest, sesame oil, and rice vinegar.

4. Spoon a small amount of turkey stuffing onto each lettuce leaf to make the lettuce wraps. Add cooked noodles and a garnish of bean sprouts,

carrots, peanuts, and cilantro on top of each.
Accompany with dipping sweet chili sauce.

4. Lentil Soup

Prep Time: 15 mins
Cook Time: 1 hr 20 mins
Total Time: 1 hr 35 mins
Servings: 8

Ingredients

- ¼ cup olive oil
- 1 onion, chopped
- 2 carrots, diced
- 2 stalks celery, chopped
- 2 cloves garlic, minced
- 1 bay leaf
- 1 teaspoon dried oregano
- 1 teaspoon dried basil

- 2 cups dry lentils
- 8 cups water
- 1 (14.5 ounce) can crushed tomatoes
- ½ cup spinach, rinsed and thinly sliced
- 2 tablespoons vinegar
- salt to taste
- ground black pepper to taste

Directions

1. In a large soup pot, heat the oil over medium heat. Add the onions, carrots, and celery; simmer and stir for 3 to 5 minutes, or until the onion is soft.

2. Cook for two minutes after adding the garlic, basil, bay leaf, and oregano.

3. Add the tomatoes and water, then stir in the lentils. Heat till boiling. Simmer the lentils for at least an hour on low heat, or until they are soft.

4. Add spinach and simmer until it wilts just before serving.

5. Mix in the vinegar and add salt and pepper to taste, adjusting as necessary.

6. Present heated and relish.

5.Chickpea Salad with Red Onion & Tomatoes

Prep Time: 10 mins
Additional Time: 2 hrs
Total Time: 2 hrs 10 mins
Servings: 4

Ingredients

- 19 ounces garbanzo beans, drained
- 2 tablespoons red onion, chopped
- 2 cloves garlic, minced
- 1 tomato, chopped
- ½ cup chopped parsley
- 3 tablespoons olive oil
- 1 tablespoon lemon juice
- salt and pepper to taste

Directions

1. Combine the chickpeas, lemon juice, olive oil, red onion, garlic, tomato, parsley, and salt and pepper to taste in a big bowl. Let cool for two hours prior to serving. Taste and modify the seasoning.
2. Present and Savor

6.Vietnamese Fresh Spring Rolls

Prep Time: 45 mins
Cook Time: 5 mins
Total Time: 50 mins
Servings: 8

Ingredients

- 2 ounces rice vermicelli
- 8 rice wrappers (8.5 inch diameter)
- 8 large cooked shrimp - peeled, deveined and cut in half
- 2 leaves lettuce, chopped
- 3 tablespoons chopped fresh mint leaves
- 3 tablespoons chopped fresh cilantro

- 1 ⅓ tablespoons chopped fresh Thai basil

Sauces

- ¼ cup water
- 2 tablespoons fresh lime juice
- 2 tablespoons white sugar
- 4 teaspoons fish sauce
- 1 clove garlic, minced
- ½ teaspoon garlic chili sauce
- 3 tablespoons hoisin sauce
- 1 teaspoon finely chopped peanuts

Directions

1. Add vermicelli noodles to a large pot of lightly salted water and bring to a rolling boil; toss and return to a boil. Cook pasta uncovered for 3 to 5 minutes, stirring regularly, or until it's firm to the bite but still soft.

2. Pour warm water into a sizable dish. To soften, dip one wrapper into the hot water for one second. Lay out the wrapper flat. Arrange the two shrimp

halves in a row across the middle. Top with the lettuce, mint, cilantro, and basil, and reserve approximately 2 inches on each side. Starting with the lettuce at the end, tightly roll the wrapper by folding the uncovered sides inside. Proceed with the remaining components.

3. For the sauces: In a small dish, thoroughly mix the water, lime juice, sugar, fish sauce, garlic, and chili sauce. In a small bowl, combine peanuts and hoisin sauce.

4. Present wrapped spring rolls accompanied by hoisin and fish sauce concoctions.

7.Mediterranean Quinoa Salad

Prep Time: 15 mins
Cook Time: 20 mins
Total Time: 35 mins
Servings: 8

Ingredients

- 2 cups water

- 2 cubes chicken bouillon
- 1 clove garlic, smashed
- 1 cup uncooked quinoa
- 2 large cooked chicken breasts - cut into bite size pieces
- 1 large red onion, diced
- 1 large green bell pepper, diced
- ½ cup chopped kalamata olives
- ½ cup crumbled feta cheese
- ¼ cup chopped fresh parsley
- ¼ cup chopped fresh chives
- ½ teaspoon salt
- ⅔ cup fresh lemon juice
- 1 tablespoon balsamic vinegar
- ¼ cup olive oil

Directions

1. In a saucepan, bring the water, bouillon cubes, and garlic to a boil. After adding the quinoa, simmer for 15 to 20 minutes, covered, over medium-low heat, or until the quinoa is soft and the water has been absorbed. Scrape the quinoa into a large basin and discard the garlic clove.

2. Carefully mix the quinoa with the chicken, onion, bell pepper, olives, feta cheese, parsley, chives, and salt. Pour in the olive oil, balsamic vinegar, and lemon juice. Mix well, stirring until combined. Serve warm or cold, straight from the refrigerator.

8.Yummy Beef Stir Fry

Prep Time: 15 mins
Cook Time: 10 mins
Total Time: 25 mins
Servings: 4

Ingredients
- 2 tablespoons vegetable oil
- 1 pound beef sirloin, cut into 2-inch strips
- 1 ½ cups fresh broccoli florets
- 1 red bell pepper, cut into matchsticks
- 2 carrots, thinly sliced

- 1 green onion, chopped
- 1 teaspoon minced garlic
- 2 tablespoons soy sauce
- 2 tablespoons sesame seeds, toasted

Directions

1. Compile all of the ingredients.

2. In a large wok or skillet over medium-high heat, heat the vegetable oil; cook and stir the meat for 3 to 4 minutes, or until browned.

3. Slide the steak to one side of the skillet and place the broccoli, carrots, bell pepper, green onion, and garlic in the middle of the wok. For two minutes, cook and stir the vegetables.

4. Stir the steak into the veggies and add sesame seeds and soy sauce for seasoning. Cook and toss the vegetables for an additional two minutes or until they are soft.

5. Present warm and savor!

9.Turkey Avocado Panini

Prep Time: 17 mins
Cook Time: 8 mins
Total Time: 25 mins
Servings: 2

Ingredients

½ ripe avocado

¼ cup mayonnaise

2 ciabatta rolls

1 tablespoon olive oil, divided

2 slices provolone cheese

1 cup whole fresh spinach leaves, divided

¼ pound thinly sliced mesquite smoked turkey breast

2 roasted red peppers, sliced into strips

Directions

1. In a bowl, mash the avocado and mayonnaise until well combined.

2. Set a panini sandwich press to preheat.

3. Divide the ciabatta buns in half lengthwise and lightly coat the underside of each roll with olive oil before assembling the sandwiches. With the olive oil side facing down, place the roll bottoms onto the panini press. Top each sandwich with a slice of provolone cheese, half the spinach leaves, half the sliced turkey breast, and a sliced roasted red pepper. Lay the top of the roll on top of the sandwich after spreading half of the avocado mixture over each top's cut surface. Drizzle a little olive oil over the roll's top.

4. Close the panini press and cook for 5 to 8 minutes, or until the cheese has melted and the bun is crisp and toasted with golden brown grill marks.

10.Baked Sweet Potato Fries

Prep Time: 10 mins

Cook Time: 20 mins
Total Time: 35 mins
Servings: 4

Ingredients

- 2 large sweet potatoes
- 3 tablespoons soybean oil (often labeled "vegetable oil")
- ½ teaspoon sea salt
- ½ teaspoon freshly ground black pepper
- ¼ teaspoon garlic powder
- ¼ teaspoon paprika

Directions

1. Compile all of the ingredients.
2. Set the oven's temperature to 425 F (220 C). Place the rack in the oven's highest third. Coat a baking sheet in oil.
3. Cut sweet potatoes into 1x3-inch wedges after peeling them. In a large dish, combine the

wedges and the soybean oil; toss lightly. Add paprika, garlic powder, salt, and pepper.

4. Spread out potatoes on the prepared baking sheet in a single layer, taking care not to pile them too close together. Bake for 18 to 24 minutes, turning regularly, or until tender and golden brown. Let it cool for five minutes before serving.

Chapter 6

Flavorful and Allergy-Safe Dinner Recipes

1.Roasted Lemon Herb Chicken

Prep Time: 15 mins
Cook Time: 1 hr 30 mins
Total Time: 1 hr 45 mins
Servings: 8.

Ingredients

- 2 teaspoons Italian seasoning
- ½ teaspoon seasoning salt

- ½ teaspoon mustard powder
- 1 teaspoon garlic powder
- ½ teaspoon ground black pepper
- 1 (3 pound) whole chicken
- 2 lemons
- 2 tablespoons olive oil

Directions

1. Set oven temperature to 350 F (175 C).

2. Mix the spices, black pepper, mustard powder, and garlic powder; put aside. After giving the chicken a good rinse, take off the giblets. Chicken should be put in a 9 x 13-inch baking dish. Inside the chicken, distribute 1 1/2 teaspoons of the spice mixture. Apply the leftover mixture on the chicken's exterior.

3. Transfer the juice from both lemons into a tiny cup or bowl and whisk in the olive oil. Over the chicken, drizzle this oil/juice mixture.

4. Bake, basting frequently with the leftover oil mixture, in the preheated oven for one and a half hours, or until juices run clear.

2.Balsamic Bruschetta

Prep Time: 15 mins
Cook Time: 5 mins
Total Time: 20 mins
Servings: 8

Ingredients

- 1 loaf French bread, cut into 1/4-inch slices
- 1 tablespoon extra-virgin olive oil
- 8 roma (plum) tomatoes, diced
- ⅓ cup chopped fresh basil
- 1 ounce Parmesan cheese, freshly grated
- 2 cloves garlic, minced
- 1 tablespoon good quality balsamic vinegar
- 2 teaspoons extra-virgin olive oil
- ¼ teaspoon kosher salt
- ¼ teaspoon freshly ground black pepper

Directions

1. Compile the ingredients.
2. Set oven temperature to 400 F, or 200 C.
3. Lightly oil both sides of the bread pieces and arrange them on a sizable baking sheet. Toast the bread for 5 to 10 minutes, flipping it halfway through, or until golden.
4. Meanwhile, combine the tomatoes, garlic, basil, and Parmesan cheese in a bowl.
5. Incorporate kosher salt, pepper, two tsp olive oil, and balsamic vinegar.
6. Spoon tomato mixture onto slices of toast.
7. Serve right away and savor!

3.cedar Planked Salmon

See how to make a tasty salmon meal with cedar planks that is ideal for children with EoE. This recipe, which is flavorful, smokey, and moist, is popular with both adults and children. For a wholesome and filling dinner, serve it with asparagus and kid-friendly Asian-style rice.

Prep Time: 15 mins
Cook Time: 20 mins
Total Time: 35 mins
Servings:.   6

Ingredients

- 3 (12 inch) untreated cedar planks
- ⅓ cup soy sauce
- ⅓ cup vegetable oil
- 1 ½ tablespoons rice vinegar
- 1 teaspoon sesame oil
- ¼ cup chopped green onions
- 1 tablespoon grated fresh ginger
- 1 teaspoon minced garlic
- 2 (2 pound) salmon filets, skin removed

Directions

1. Soak cedar boards in warm water for a minimum of one hour. If you have time, continue to soak.

2. In a shallow dish, combine soy sauce, vegetable oil, rice vinegar, sesame oil, green onions, ginger, and garlic.

3. After adding the soy mixture, turn the salmon filets to coat. For a minimum of fifteen minutes, or up to an hour if refrigerated, cover and marinate.

4. Set an outside grill to a medium temperature. Organize the barbecue grate using planks. Preheat the boards until they begin to smoke and crackle slightly.

5.Discard marinade and arrange salmon on planks after removing it from the marinade.

6. Shut the grill lid. About 20 minutes of grilling is enough to make salmon flake easily with a fork; the salmon will continue to cook after you take it from the grill.

4. Quinoa Stuffed Peppers

Prep Time: 30 mins
Cook Time: 50 mins
Total Time: 1 hr 20 mins
Servings: 6

Ingredients

- 1 cup quinoa, rinsed and drained
- 2 cups water
- 2 tablespoons olive oil
- 1 small onion, diced
- 2 cloves garlic, minced
- 1 zucchini, diced
- 1 small eggplant, diced
- 1 tomato, diced
- 1 cup tomato sauce
- salt and ground black pepper to taste
- 6 bell peppers, tops cut off and seeded
- 1 cup shredded mozzarella cheese, or more to taste

Directions

1. Set oven temperature to 350 F (175 C). Line a baking dish that is deep with aluminum foil.

2. In a saucepan, combine the quinoa and water; bring to a boil. After the quinoa is soft and the water has been absorbed, cover, lower the heat, and simmer for about 15 minutes.

3. In a large skillet over medium heat, heat the olive oil; sauté and toss the onion and garlic for 5 to 7 minutes, or until aromatic and beginning to turn translucent. Cook for 3 to 5 minutes, or until the zucchini, eggplant, and tomato are slightly soft. Mix tomato sauce with vegetable mixture; cover and cook for an additional 10 minutes or until veggies are tender.

4. Add quinoa to the mixture of vegetables. Add pepper and salt for seasoning. Pack the quinoa-vegetable mixture into bell peppers. Put peppers in a baking dish that has been ready. Wrap the dish in aluminum foil.

5. Bake for about 18 minutes, or until the bell peppers are just starting to soften, in a preheated oven. Take off the aluminum foil cover and add mozzarella cheese to the peppers. Bake for a further five minutes or until the cheese is melted and bubbling.

5.Ratatouille

Prep Time: 15 mins

Cook Time: 45 mins
Total Time: 1 hr
Servings: 4

Ingredients

- 2 tablespoons olive oil, divided
- 3 cloves garlic, minced
- 1 eggplant, cut into 1/2 inch cubes
- 2 teaspoons dried parsley
- salt to taste
- 1 cup grated Parmesan cheese
- 2 zucchini, sliced
- 2 large tomatoes, chopped
- 2 cups sliced fresh mushrooms
- 1 large onion, sliced into rings
- 1 green or red bell pepper, sliced

Directions

1. Set the oven's temperature to 350°F, or 175°C. Grease a 1-1/2-quart casserole dish from bottom to side with one tablespoon of olive oil.

2. In a medium skillet, preheat the final tablespoon of olive oil over medium heat. Garlic is cooked and stirred until aromatic and golden brown. After adding the eggplant and parsley, heat and stir for ten minutes or until the eggplant is soft and tender. Add salt to taste to season.

3. Evenly distribute the eggplant mixture in the bottom of the casserole dish that has been prepared, and top with a few tablespoons of Parmesan cheese. Evenly distribute the zucchini on top. Season with a little salt and add a bit extra cheese. Continue layering in this manner with the bell pepper, onion, mushrooms, and tomatoes, finishing each layer with a sprinkle of cheese and salt.

4. Bake for 45 minutes or until the vegetables are soft in a preheated oven.

Chapter 7

Sweet Treats: Desserts Without the EOE Worry

1.Fruit Skewers

Prep Time: 15 mins
Total Time: 15 mins
Servings: 5

Ingredients

- 5 large strawberries, halved
- ¼ cantaloupe, cut into balls or cubes

- 2 bananas, peeled and cut into chunks
- 1 medium apple, cut into chunks
- 20 skewers

Directions

1. Thread pieces of apple, banana, cantaloupe, and strawberry alternately onto skewers; skewers should have a minimum of two pieces of fruit each. Skewers should be arranged artistically on a serving dish.

2.Mango Sticky Rice

Prep Time: 10 mins
Total Time: 1 hr 30 mins
Servings: 4

Ingredients.

- 2 cups water
- 1 ½ cups uncooked short-grain white rice

- 1 ½ cups coconut milk, divided
- 1 cup white sugar
- ¾ teaspoon salt, divided
- 1 tablespoon white sugar
- 1 tablespoon tapioca starch
- 3 mangos, peeled and sliced
- 1 tablespoon toasted sesame seeds

Directions.

1. Fill a saucepan with rice and water. After bringing to a boil, lower heat and cover. Simmer for 15 to 20 minutes, or until water is absorbed.
2. Transfer 1 1/2 cups coconut milk, 1 cup sugar, and 1/2 teaspoon salt to another skillet and heat while the rice cooks. Over medium heat, bring to a boil; take off and put aside.
3. Mix the cooked rice with the mixture of coconut milk. After covering, give it an hour to cool.
4. In a separate pot, make the sauce by mixing 1/2 cup coconut milk, 1 tablespoon sugar, 1/4 teaspoon salt, and tapioca starch. Bring to a boil.

5. Transfer the coconut rice to a platter and top with the mangos. Drizzle rice and mangos with sauce. Add sesame seeds on top.

3.Warm Berry Compote

Prep Time: 5 mins
Cook Time: 1 hr 40 mins
Total Time: 1 hr 45 mins
Servings: 6

Ingredients

- 6 cups frozen mixed berries
- ½ cup white sugar
- ¼ cup orange juice
- 1 ½ teaspoons finely grated orange zest
- 2 tablespoons cornstarch
- 2 tablespoons water

Directions

1. In a slow cooker, combine sugar, orange juice, zest, and frozen berries. Once bubbling, cover and simmer on High for approximately 1 1/2 hours.

2. In a cup, whisk together cornstarch and water until completely dissolved. Add to the fruit mixture and stir. Cook, covered again, for 5 to 10 minutes, or until thickened. Heat or serve room temperature.

4.Pina Colada Sorbet

Prep Time: 25 min
Total Time: 25 mins
Servings: 9

Ingredients

- 1 ½ cups white sugar
- 1 ½ cups water
- 1 (20 ounce) can canned crushed pineapple, drained
- 1 (13.5 ounce) can coconut milk
- ¼ cup lime juice

Directions

1. To make a syrup, place the sugar and water in a small saucepan over high heat. Stir and boil, covered, for one minute or until the liquid turns clear. Put aside to cool.

2. Using a blender or food processor, puree the drained pineapple until it becomes extremely smooth and frothy. Mix the syrup, lime juice, coconut milk, and pineapple puree in a big bowl. Put in the fridge for three hours or until cooled.

3.Freeze in the ice cream maker's freezer canister per the manufacturer's instructions.

5.Watermelon Mojito Granita

Prep Time: 10 mins
Additional Time: 4 hrs
Total Time: 4 hrs 10 mins
Servings: 5

Ingredients

- 1 small seedless watermelon
- 1 cup water
- ½ cup white sugar
- 3 leaves fresh mint
- ⅓ cup white rum

Directions

1. Slice the watermelon into large chunks after removing the rind. In an electric blender, combine watermelon, sugar, mint leaves, and water. Puree in a blender.

2.Add the rum and swirl a few times to mix it in. After filling a 9 by 12 pan, transfer the mixture there and freeze for four hours. Every one to two hours, scrape the mixture with a fork. Because of the rum, it will not freeze fully.

3. Present in a pretty glass or a shallow dish.

6.Frozen Banana Bites

Prep Time: 30 mins
Cooking Time: 1 hr 45 mins
Total Time: 2 hrs 15 mins
Servings: 45

Ingredients

- 1 cup peanut butter
- 4 bananas, sliced into 1-inch rounds
- 8 (1 ounce) squares semisweet chocolate
- 1 tablespoon shortening
- ⅓ cup toffee baking bits

Directions

1. Use wax paper to cover a baking sheet.

2. Top each slice of banana with a small dollop of peanut butter. Take a toothpick and poke it through the banana's peanut butter coating. Put the banana bites on the baking sheet that has been prepared, and freeze for 30 to 60 minutes.

3. In a double boiler set over simmering water, melt the shortening and chocolate, stirring often and

scraping down the sides with a rubber spatula to prevent burning.

4. Use wax paper to cover an additional baking sheet.

5. Take out two to four bites of banana from the freezer at a time, and then cover each mouthful with chocolate mixture. Scatter toffee bits over each covered banana bite before placing them on the second baking sheet. Continue until all of the bites have a coating. Place banana bites back in the freezer for at least one hour to solidify. Before serving, let the bites remain at room temperature for approximately fifteen minutes.

Chapter 8

Managing Eosinophilic Esophagitis Beyond Diet

There is undoubtedly more to treating Eosinophilic Esophagitis (EoE) in children than merely monitoring their food. Let's examine some essential ideas that can offer a thorough strategy for successfully controlling this illness.

1. Medication Management: To assist reduce inflammation and symptoms, it's critical to collaborate closely with your child's doctor to identify the appropriate drugs. Mast cell stabilizers, ingested steroids, and proton pump inhibitors (PPIs) are common choices.

2. Allergy Testing: An important factor in EoE is frequently allergies. Testing can assist in identifying certain triggers, such as environmental variables or dietary allergies, enabling the development of focused avoidance tactics.

3. Observing Symptoms: Maintaining a symptom journal can give important information about possible triggers and the efficacy of treatment. Record the symptoms, when they happen, how severe they are, and any trends you see.

4. Follow-up Endoscopies: To evaluate therapy response, track inflammation levels, and modify the management strategy as necessary, periodic endoscopies may be advised.

5. Behavioral and Emotional Support: It can be difficult for children to live with a chronic illness like EoE. For their general wellbeing, it is essential to offer them emotional support and guide them through any social or psychological challenges.

6. Nutritional Support: Consulting with a dietician can help you manage food limitations and make sure your child is getting enough nourishment. It could be required to take supplements or eat different foods to keep a balanced diet.

7.Educating Teachers and Other Caregivers: To protect your child's safety and wellbeing when they're not from home, it's critical to inform teachers, other caregivers, and school personnel about EoE, how it's managed, and any necessary dietary restrictions or emergency protocols.

8. Joining Support Groups: Making connections with other families dealing with comparable issues can provide priceless resources, support, and insights. Local community groups, online forums, and support groups can all be excellent places to get advice and assistance.